OPTIMIZE YOUR HEALTH

The Ultimate Guide to Lowering High Triglycerides with a Targeted Diet Plan

Adams .U. Morris

TABLE OF CONTENTS

CHAPTER 1

High Triglycerides diet

In the world of health and nutrition, the term "triglycerides" often gets thrown around, but what exactly are they, and why should we care about them? Chapter 1 of our book, "Taming Triglycerides," sets the stage by diving deep into the fundamentals of triglycerides, shedding light on their role in the body, defining what high triglycerides are, and illuminating the connection between elevated triglyceride levels and our cardiovascular health.

The Basics of Triglycerides

Triglycerides are a type of fat (lipid) found in your blood. They're a fundamental component of the body's energy storage system, serving as a primary source of energy. When you eat, your body converts the excess calories into triglycerides, which are then stored in fat cells. Later, when your body needs energy, these triglycerides are released into the bloodstream and broken down for fuel.

The Role of Triglycerides

Now, let's talk about why triglycerides are essential. In their rightful place and quantity, triglycerides are essential for our health. They provide energy to our muscles, helping us perform physical activities, and they're also stored as fat for later use. They're like the energy savings account of our bodies.

The Connection Between Triglycerides and Cardiovascular Health

High triglyceride levels, on the other hand, can spell trouble for your heart and overall health. Elevated triglycerides have been linked to a higher risk of cardiovascular diseases, including heart attacks and strokes. When triglycerides are excessively high, they can contribute to the formation of arterial plaque, which narrows and hardens the arteries. This can obstruct blood flow and increase the risk of heart disease.

Identifying High Triglycerides

So, how do you know if you have high triglycerides? A standard blood test can measure your triglyceride levels. The results are usually reported in milligrams per deciliter (mg/dL) of blood. Here's how the American Heart Association classifies triglyceride levels:

- Normal: Less than 150 mg/dL
- Borderline high: 150-199 mg/dL
- High: 200-499 mg/dL
- Very high: 500 mg/dL or above

If your levels fall into the "high" or "very high" categories, it's essential to take action to lower them and reduce your risk of cardiovascular disease.

Causes and Risk Factors for Elevated Triglycerides

High triglycerides can result from various factors, including genetics, diet, lifestyle, and underlying medical conditions. Some common risk factors for elevated triglycerides include:

1. **Diet:** A diet high in sugar, refined carbohydrates, and unhealthy fats (such as saturated and trans fats) can contribute to high triglycerides. Excessive alcohol consumption can also elevate triglyceride levels.

2. **Obesity:** Being overweight or obese is often associated with higher triglycerides. Fat cells not only store excess energy as triglycerides but can also release them into the bloodstream.

3. **Physical Inactivity:** A sedentary lifestyle can lead to elevated triglycerides. Regular physical activity helps your body use triglycerides for energy and lowers their levels in the bloodstream.

4. **Genetics:** Some people may inherit a genetic predisposition to high

triglycerides. This condition, called familial hypertriglyceridemia, can lead to very high triglyceride levels.

5. **Medical Conditions:** Certain medical conditions, such as type 2 diabetes, metabolic syndrome, and polycystic ovary syndrome (PCOS), are associated with elevated triglycerides.

6. **Medications:** Some medications, like certain steroids, diuretics, and beta-blockers, can raise triglyceride levels as a side effect.

7. **Other Lifestyle Factors:** Smoking and stress can also impact triglyceride levels indirectly by affecting eating habits and overall health.

The Big Picture

Chapter 1 aims to establish a solid foundation of knowledge about triglycerides. We've learned that these fatty molecules play a crucial role in our bodies, serving as a source of energy and being stored as fat for later use. However, when triglyceride levels become too high, they can pose a significant risk to our cardiovascular health.

By understanding what triglycerides are, how they function, and the factors that contribute to elevated levels, you're better equipped to tackle the issue. The chapter also serves as a wakeup call, emphasizing the importance of regular check-ups and blood tests to monitor your triglyceride levels, especially if you have risk factors like a family history of heart disease or obesity.

In the chapters that follow, we'll explore dietary and lifestyle changes you can make to manage and lower your triglyceride levels. Armed with this knowledge, you can take proactive steps to protect your heart and overall well-being. So, let's move forward in our journey toward a healthier, triglyceride-friendly diet.

CHAPTER 2

The Basics of a Triglyceride-Friendly Diet

In Chapter 1, we laid the foundation for understanding triglycerides and why they matter for your health. Now, in Chapter 2, we're delving into the heart of the matter – what constitutes a triglyceride-friendly diet? This chapter will explore the fundamental principles of such a diet, emphasizing the importance of calories, macronutrients, portion control, balanced meals, and regular eating patterns.

Calories and Triglycerides

Calories are units of energy derived from the foods and beverages we consume. It's important to recognize that excess calorie intake plays a pivotal role in triglyceride levels. When you consume more calories than your body needs, these excess calories are converted into triglycerides and stored as fat. Over time, this can lead to elevated triglyceride levels.

Portion Control

Portion control is a vital aspect of managing calorie intake and, consequently, triglyceride levels. It's easy to underestimate portion sizes in today's super-sized culture. Paying attention to portion sizes can help you avoid overeating and the resulting excess calories.

To practice portion control:

- Use smaller plates and bowls to encourage smaller portions.
- Read food labels to understand serving sizes.
- Learn to estimate portion sizes visually.

- Avoid "all-you-can-eat" buffets, which can encourage overeating.

Balanced Meals

Balanced meals are key to a triglyceride-friendly diet. A balanced meal typically includes a mix of carbohydrates, protein, and healthy fats. This combination provides sustained energy, promotes satiety, and helps regulate blood sugar levels, all of which can aid in controlling triglycerides.

Regular Eating Patterns

Establishing regular eating patterns can also help stabilize triglyceride levels. Irregular eating habits, such as skipping meals or going long periods without food, can lead to fluctuations in blood sugar levels. These fluctuations can trigger the release of triglycerides into the bloodstream.

To establish regular eating patterns:

- Aim for three balanced meals each day.
- Include healthy snacks if needed to avoid prolonged periods without eating.

- Try to eat meals and snacks at consistent times.

The Glycemic Index

In addition to considering calories and portion control, understanding the glycemic index (GI) can be beneficial for managing triglycerides. The GI is a scale that measures how quickly carbohydrates in foods raise blood sugar levels. Foods with a high GI cause rapid spikes and crashes in blood sugar, which can influence triglyceride levels.

Foods with a low GI, on the other hand, cause a slower, more gradual increase in blood sugar. This can help maintain stable triglyceride levels and reduce the risk of overeating due to sudden hunger.

Putting It All Together

So, what does a typical triglyceride-friendly meal look like? Let's put these principles into action:

1. **Carbohydrates:** Choose complex carbohydrates like whole grains (brown rice, quinoa, whole wheat bread), legumes (beans, lentils), and non-starchy vegetables

(broccoli, spinach). These foods have a lower GI and provide sustained energy.

2. **Protein:** Include lean sources of protein such as skinless poultry, fish, tofu, and beans. Protein helps you feel full and satisfied, reducing the likelihood of overeating.

3. **Healthy Fats:** Incorporate sources of healthy fats like avocados, nuts, seeds, and olive oil. These fats provide essential nutrients and can help stabilize blood sugar.

4. **Portion Control:** Pay attention to portion sizes. A

typical plate might consist of half non-starchy vegetables, a quarter lean protein, and a quarter whole grains.

5. **Regular Eating Patterns:** Aim to eat at regular intervals throughout the day, such as breakfast, lunch, dinner, and healthy snacks in between if needed.

6. **Hydration:** Stay hydrated with water or unsweetened beverages. Dehydration can sometimes lead to overeating or cravings.

The Big Picture

In Chapter 2, we've explored the core elements of a triglyceride-friendly diet: calories, portion control, balanced meals, regular eating patterns, and the glycemic index. These principles provide a solid framework for making informed dietary choices that can help you manage and lower your triglyceride levels.

The key takeaway is that a healthy diet is not just about what you eat but also about how much you eat and when you eat it. By paying attention to these factors and making conscious choices, you can take significant steps toward achieving and maintaining healthy triglyceride levels.

In the chapters that follow, we'll delve deeper into specific aspects of your diet, such as the types of fats and carbohydrates you should prioritize, and we'll provide practical tips and meal ideas to help you put these principles into practice. Remember, the journey to taming your triglycerides is about making sustainable, positive changes to your eating habits, and Chapter 2 is your starting point on this path to better health.

CHAPTER 3

Choosing the Right Fats

In Chapter 2, we laid the foundation for a triglyceride-friendly diet by discussing the importance of calories, portion control, balanced meals, and regular eating patterns. Now, in Chapter 3, we dive deeper into a critical aspect of this dietary journey—fats. We'll explore the various types of dietary fats and their impact on triglyceride levels, emphasizing the importance of choosing the right fats for a heart-healthy lifestyle.

The Different Types of Dietary Fats

Not all fats are created equal, and understanding the distinctions between different types of dietary fats is crucial for managing triglycerides. Dietary fats can be broadly categorized into three main types:

1. **Saturated Fats:** These fats are typically solid at room temperature and are commonly found in animal-based products such as fatty

cuts of meat, full-fat dairy products, and certain tropical oils like coconut and palm oil. Consuming too much saturated fat can increase both triglyceride levels and LDL (low-density lipoprotein) cholesterol, which is often referred to as "bad" cholesterol.

2. **Trans Fats:** Trans fats are artificial fats created through a process called hydrogenation. They were once commonly used in processed foods to extend shelf life and improve texture. However, trans fats

are strongly associated with heart disease and should be avoided as much as possible. Thankfully, many countries have banned or significantly reduced their use in food products.

3. **Unsaturated Fats:** These are the healthy fats you want to include in your diet. Unsaturated fats can be further divided into two categories:

    o **Monounsaturated Fats:** Found in foods like olive oil, avocados, nuts (especially almonds and cashews), and seeds, monounsaturated fats have been shown to improve blood lipid profiles, including reducing triglycerides.

- **Polyunsaturated Fats:** These fats are found in fatty fish (like salmon, mackerel, and trout), flaxseeds, walnuts, and certain vegetable oils (such as soybean and corn oil). They are particularly rich in essential omega-3 and omega-6 fatty acids, which have

various health
benefits, including
reducing inflammation
and lowering
triglyceride levels.

The Role of Healthy Fats in Triglyceride Management

Now that we've identified the good fats (unsaturated fats) and the fats to avoid (saturated and trans fats), let's explore how incorporating healthy fats into your diet can contribute to triglyceride management:

1. **Omega-3 Fatty Acids:** These are a type of

polyunsaturated fat found in fatty fish and some plant-based sources like flaxseeds and walnuts. Omega-3s have been shown to lower triglyceride levels, reduce inflammation, and support overall heart health.

2. **Monounsaturated Fats:** Foods rich in monounsaturated fats, such as olive oil and avocados, can improve your blood lipid profile, including lowering triglycerides.

3. **Replacing Saturated and Trans Fats:** One of the most effective ways to lower

triglyceride levels is to replace saturated and trans fats in your diet with unsaturated fats. For example, you can switch from butter (saturated fat) to olive oil (monounsaturated fat) for cooking or from deep-fried foods (often containing trans fats) to grilled fish (rich in omega-3s).

Practical Tips for Incorporating Healthy Fats

Now that we've discussed the importance of healthy fats, let's explore some practical tips for incorporating them into your diet:

1. **Cook with Olive Oil:** Replace butter or lard with olive oil when sautéing or frying foods. Olive oil is rich in heart-healthy monounsaturated fats.

2. **Add Nuts and Seeds:** Sprinkle chopped nuts (like almonds or walnuts) and seeds (such as flaxseeds or chia seeds) on salads, yogurt, or oatmeal. They provide healthy fats and added texture and flavor.

3. **Eat Fatty Fish:** Aim to include fatty fish like salmon, mackerel, or sardines in your diet at least twice a week. These fish are excellent sources of omega-3 fatty acids.

4. **Snack Smart:** Choose snacks like unsalted nuts, trail mix with dried fruits, or sliced avocado on whole-grain crackers. These options provide healthy fats and can help you stay satisfied between meals.

5. **Avocado Love:** Avocado is not only delicious but also a great source of

monounsaturated fats. Mash it for guacamole, slice it for sandwiches, or spread it on whole-grain toast.

6. **Read Food Labels:** When shopping for packaged foods, check the nutrition labels for information on saturated and trans fats. Aim for products with minimal or zero trans fats and limited saturated fat content.

Balancing Fats in Your Diet

While incorporating healthy fats is crucial, it's essential to maintain a balanced diet overall. A triglyceride-friendly diet doesn't mean avoiding all fats but rather choosing the right fats in the right amounts. Remember that fats are calorie-dense, so portion control remains important.

A balanced meal might consist of a moderate portion of lean protein (like grilled chicken breast or tofu), a generous serving of vegetables, and a small drizzle of olive oil for added flavor and healthy fat. By balancing your plate and making thoughtful choices, you can support your triglyceride management goals while enjoying delicious and satisfying meals.

The Big Picture

In Chapter 3, we've explored the significance of choosing the right fats for a heart-healthy, triglyceride-friendly diet. By understanding the different types of dietary fats and their impact on triglycerides, you're equipped to make informed choices when it comes to meal planning and food selection. Incorporating healthy fats, such as omega-3s, monounsaturated fats, and polyunsaturated fats, can be a powerful tool in your journey to taming triglycerides.

The key takeaway is that fats are not your enemy; it's about choosing the right fats and consuming them in appropriate quantities. By doing so, you'll not only support your triglyceride management but also promote overall cardiovascular health and well-being. In the chapters that follow, we'll continue to explore dietary strategies and practical tips to help you achieve and maintain healthy triglyceride levels.

CHAPTER 4

Carbohydrates and Triglycerides

As we journey through our exploration of taming high triglycerides with a healthy diet, we arrive at Chapter 4, where we delve into the often-misunderstood world of carbohydrates. Carbohydrates are a staple in most diets, and they play a significant role in our overall health. In this chapter, we'll explore the relationship between carbohydrates and triglycerides, focusing on how the type and quantity of carbs you consume can impact your triglyceride levels.

Understanding Carbohydrates

Carbohydrates are one of the three essential macronutrients, along with proteins and fats. They are the body's primary source of energy. Carbohydrates are found in various foods, including grains, fruits, vegetables, legumes, and dairy products. They come in two main forms:

1. **Complex Carbohydrates:**
   These are made up of long chains of sugar molecules and are found in foods like whole grains (brown rice, whole wheat bread, quinoa), starchy vegetables (potatoes, sweet potatoes), and legumes (beans, lentils). Complex carbs are rich in fiber, which helps regulate blood sugar and keeps you feeling full.

2. **Simple Carbohydrates:**
   These are composed of one or two sugar molecules and are found in foods like table sugar, candy, soda, and

many processed foods. Simple carbs are often referred to as "simple sugars" and can cause rapid spikes in blood sugar levels.

Carbohydrates and Triglycerides

The relationship between carbohydrates and triglycerides is complex but essential to understand for effective triglyceride management:

1. **The Glycemic Index (GI):** The GI is a scale that ranks carbohydrate-containing foods based on

how quickly they raise blood sugar levels. Foods with a high GI cause rapid spikes in blood sugar, while those with a low GI lead to slower, more gradual increases.

2. **High-GI Foods:** Consuming foods with a high GI can lead to elevated triglyceride levels. These foods cause spikes in blood sugar, prompting the release of insulin, a hormone that can promote triglyceride production and storage.

3. **Low-GI Foods:** On the other hand, choosing foods with a low GI can help

stabilize blood sugar levels and reduce the risk of triglyceride spikes. These foods are often high in fiber, which slows down the digestion and absorption of carbohydrates.

Balancing Carbohydrates for Triglyceride Management

Balancing carbohydrates in your diet is essential for managing triglycerides effectively. Here's how you can achieve this balance:

1. **Choose Complex Carbohydrates:** Opt for complex carbs like whole

grains, legumes, and non-starchy vegetables. These foods have a lower GI and provide sustained energy without causing rapid blood sugar spikes.

2. **Fiber Matters:** Aim to include fiber-rich foods in your meals. Fiber not only slows down the digestion of carbohydrates but also helps you feel full and satisfied, reducing the temptation to overeat.

3. **Limit Sugary Foods and Drinks:** Minimize your intake of sugary snacks, candies, sugary drinks, and

desserts. These items are typically high in simple carbohydrates and can lead to blood sugar and triglyceride spikes.

4. **Watch Your Portions:** Be mindful of portion sizes, especially when consuming carbohydrate-rich foods. Even healthy carbohydrates can contribute to elevated triglycerides if consumed in excess.

5. **Balanced Meals:** Create balanced meals that include a combination of carbohydrates, lean protein, and healthy fats. This

balance can help stabilize blood sugar levels and reduce triglyceride fluctuations.

6. **Regular Eating Patterns:** Maintain regular eating patterns with scheduled meals and snacks. Skipping meals or going long periods without food can lead to imbalanced blood sugar levels and potential triglyceride issues.

The Role of Fiber

Fiber-rich foods are particularly important in managing triglycerides. Soluble fiber, in particular, has been shown to lower triglyceride levels. Foods high in soluble fiber include oats, beans, lentils, apples, citrus fruits, and barley. By including these foods in your diet, you can help regulate blood sugar and reduce triglycerides.

Making Smart Carbohydrate Choices

To make smart carbohydrate choices for triglyceride management, consider these practical tips:

1. **Whole Grains:** Choose whole grains over refined

grains whenever possible. Whole grains are higher in fiber and nutrients and have a lower GI.

2. **Colorful Vegetables:** Load up on colorful, non-starchy vegetables like leafy greens, peppers, and broccoli. They're low in calories and carbs but rich in fiber and nutrients.

3. **Legumes:** Incorporate beans, lentils, and chickpeas into your diet. They're excellent sources of fiber and plant-based protein.

4. **Portion Control:** Be mindful of portion sizes,

especially with carbohydrate-rich foods. Use measuring cups or your hand as a guide to appropriate portions.

5. **Low-GI Fruits:** Opt for low-GI fruits like berries, cherries, and apples. These fruits provide natural sweetness without causing rapid blood sugar spikes.

The Big Picture

In Chapter 4, we've explored the intricate relationship between carbohydrates and triglycerides. Understanding the difference between complex and simple carbohydrates and their impact on blood sugar levels is essential for managing and taming high triglycerides. By making informed choices and balancing your carbohydrate intake with fiber-rich, low-GI foods, you can help stabilize blood sugar and reduce triglyceride fluctuations.

As we move forward in our journey toward a triglyceride-friendly diet, remember that carbohydrates are not the enemy; it's about making wise choices and maintaining a balanced approach to your overall nutrition. In the chapters that follow, we'll continue to uncover dietary strategies and practical tips to help you achieve and maintain healthy triglyceride levels, one meal at a time.

CHAPTER 5

Protein and Triglycerides

Welcome to Chapter 5 of "Taming Triglycerides." We've navigated through essential aspects of a triglyceride-friendly diet, including fats and carbohydrates. Now, it's time to turn our attention to another critical macronutrient: protein. This chapter delves into the role of protein in managing triglycerides, explores sources of lean protein, addresses portion control, and emphasizes the importance of balancing protein intake with other macronutrients.

The Importance of Protein

Protein is a fundamental building block for your body. It plays a vital role in many physiological processes, including tissue repair, immune function, enzyme production, and muscle maintenance. Protein also contributes to feelings of fullness and satiety, making it an important component of a balanced meal.

Protein and Triglycerides

Protein intake can influence triglyceride levels in several ways:

1. **Satiety:** Protein-rich foods can help you feel full and satisfied, which may reduce the temptation to overeat and contribute to better overall calorie control.

2. **Muscle Maintenance:** Protein is essential for maintaining and repairing muscle tissue. Muscle tissue burns calories, so preserving lean muscle mass can support a healthy metabolism.

3. **Reducing High-Glycemic Carbohydrates:** When protein is included in a meal, it can help stabilize blood sugar levels by slowing the absorption of carbohydrates. This can indirectly support triglyceride management, as high-glycemic carbohydrates are associated with triglyceride spikes.

Choosing Lean Protein Sources

Not all protein sources are created equal. To keep your triglycerides in check, it's important to choose lean sources of protein that are lower in saturated fat. Here are some examples:

1. **Poultry:** Skinless poultry, such as chicken and turkey, is a lean source of protein. Remove the skin to reduce saturated fat content further.

2. **Fish:** Fatty fish like salmon, mackerel, and trout are not only high in protein but also rich in heart-healthy omega-3 fatty acids.

3. **Plant-Based Proteins:** Beans, lentils, tofu, tempeh, and edamame are excellent sources of plant-based protein. They are low in

saturated fat and provide fiber, which supports overall heart health.

4. **Lean Cuts of Meat:** If you prefer red meat, opt for lean cuts like sirloin, tenderloin, or loin chops. Trim visible fat before cooking.

5. **Dairy:** Low-fat or fat-free dairy products, such as yogurt, milk, and cottage cheese, offer protein without excessive saturated fat.

6. **Eggs:** Eggs are a versatile source of protein. While they contain cholesterol, current dietary guidelines suggest that they can be part of a

heart-healthy diet for most people.

Portion Control with Protein

While protein is essential, portion control is equally important. Consuming more protein than your body needs can lead to an excess of calories, which may contribute to weight gain and, in turn, elevated triglycerides. Here are some guidelines for managing portion sizes:

1. **Balance Your Plate:** Aim to fill about a quarter of your plate with a protein source. The remaining space can be

allocated to vegetables, whole grains, and healthy fats.

2. **Serving Sizes:** Learn to recognize appropriate protein portion sizes. For example, a 3-ounce portion of cooked meat is roughly the size of a deck of cards.

3. **Mindful Eating:** Pay attention to your body's hunger cues. Eating slowly and savoring each bite can help you recognize when you're full and avoid overeating.

4. **Protein at Snacks:** Include protein-rich snacks

in your day to help maintain satiety between meals. Examples include Greek yogurt, a handful of nuts, or a piece of string cheese.

Balancing Protein with Other Macronutrients

While protein is a crucial component of your diet, it should be balanced with carbohydrates and fats to create well-rounded, satisfying meals. Here's how you can achieve this balance:

1. **Complex Carbohydrates:** Choose complex carbohydrates like whole

grains, vegetables, and legumes to complement your protein sources. These carbs provide fiber and sustained energy.

2. **Healthy Fats:** Include sources of healthy fats, such as avocados, nuts, seeds, and olive oil, to round out your meals. Healthy fats provide essential nutrients and help you feel satisfied.

3. **Portion Planning:** Use portion planning to create balanced meals. For instance, a balanced meal might consist of a serving of grilled chicken (protein), a

generous portion of mixed vegetables (carbohydrates and fiber), and a drizzle of olive oil (healthy fats).

4. **Hydration:** Don't forget to stay hydrated with water or other unsweetened beverages. Proper hydration is essential for overall health and digestion.

The Big Picture

Chapter 5 reinforces the importance of protein in a triglyceride-friendly diet and highlights the role of lean protein sources in managing and taming high triglycerides. By choosing lean protein options, practicing portion control, and balancing protein intake with carbohydrates and fats, you can create meals that not only support your triglyceride management goals but also contribute to overall health and well-being.

As we move forward in our exploration, remember that achieving and maintaining healthy triglyceride levels is about making informed choices, adopting sustainable eating habits, and finding a balance that works for you. In the chapters ahead, we'll continue to uncover dietary strategies and practical tips to help you on your journey to better heart health.

CHAPTER 6

Fiber and Heart Health

In our journey to tame high triglycerides with a heart-healthy diet, Chapter 6 brings us to an essential topic – dietary fiber. Fiber is often underappreciated, but it plays a crucial role in promoting heart health and managing triglyceride levels. This chapter explores the types of dietary fiber, their effects on cholesterol and triglycerides, and how to incorporate fiber-rich foods into your diet.

Understanding Dietary Fiber

Dietary fiber is a type of carbohydrate found in plant-based foods, such as fruits, vegetables, grains, legumes, nuts, and seeds. Unlike other carbohydrates, fiber isn't digested or absorbed by the body. Instead, it passes through the digestive system mostly intact, providing a range of health benefits.

Types of Dietary Fiber

Dietary fiber can be categorized into two main types:

1. **Soluble Fiber:** This type of fiber dissolves in water to

form a gel-like substance in the digestive tract. Soluble fiber is known for its cholesterol-lowering effects and its role in stabilizing blood sugar levels. It's found in foods like oats, barley, beans, lentils, fruits (especially citrus fruits), and vegetables.

2. **Insoluble Fiber:** Insoluble fiber does not dissolve in water and adds bulk to stool, promoting regular bowel movements. While it doesn't directly impact cholesterol, it contributes to digestive health and can help with

weight management. Insoluble fiber is found in whole grains, vegetables, and wheat bran.

Fiber and Triglycerides

Now, let's explore how dietary fiber can influence triglyceride levels:

1. **Soluble Fiber and Triglycerides:** Soluble fiber has been shown to reduce triglyceride levels by slowing down the absorption of dietary fats and sugars. When you consume soluble fiber-rich foods, they form a

gel in the digestive tract, which can trap some of the dietary fats and sugars, preventing them from being absorbed into the bloodstream. This can lead to lower triglyceride levels over time.

2. **Insoluble Fiber and Triglycerides:** While insoluble fiber doesn't have a direct impact on triglycerides, it plays a crucial role in overall heart health. By promoting regular bowel movements and supporting weight management, insoluble fiber

indirectly contributes to better triglyceride management.

Incorporating Fiber into Your Diet

Increasing your fiber intake can be a powerful tool for managing triglycerides and supporting heart health. Here are some practical tips for incorporating more fiber into your diet:

1. **Choose Whole Grains:** Opt for whole grains like brown rice, whole wheat pasta, quinoa, and whole-

grain bread instead of refined grains.

2. **Eat Plenty of Fruits and Vegetables:** Aim to fill half your plate with vegetables and fruits at each meal. Include a variety of colorful options to maximize nutrient intake.

3. **Add Legumes:** Beans, lentils, and chickpeas are excellent sources of fiber and plant-based protein. Use them in soups, salads, and stews.

4. **Snack on Nuts and Seeds:** A small handful of nuts or seeds makes for a

satisfying and fiber-rich snack.

5. **Use Whole Ingredients:** When cooking or baking, choose whole ingredients whenever possible. For example, use whole apples instead of applesauce or whole oats instead of instant oatmeal.

6. **Read Labels:** When shopping for packaged foods, read nutrition labels to identify products that are high in fiber and low in added sugars.

7. **Gradual Changes:** If you're not used to a high-

fiber diet, make changes gradually to avoid digestive discomfort. Increase your fiber intake slowly and drink plenty of water to aid digestion.

Meal Planning with Fiber in Mind

Creating balanced meals that include fiber-rich foods is a key strategy for managing triglycerides. Here's a simple formula to help you build fiber-rich meals:

1. **Start with Vegetables:** Fill half your plate with a

variety of colorful vegetables. They're low in calories and high in fiber and nutrients.

2. **Add Lean Protein:** Include a serving of lean protein, such as grilled chicken, fish, or beans, to help you feel full and satisfied.

3. **Choose Whole Grains:** Opt for whole grains like brown rice, quinoa, or whole wheat pasta as your carbohydrate source. These grains are rich in fiber and provide sustained energy.

4. **Healthy Fats:** Incorporate sources of healthy fats, like avocados, nuts, or olive oil, for added flavor and satiety.

5. **Don't Forget Fruit:** Finish your meal with a piece of fresh fruit or a serving of berries for dessert.

The Big Picture

Chapter 6 has shone a spotlight on the often-overlooked hero of heart health – dietary fiber. Understanding the two main types of fiber, soluble and insoluble, and how they can impact triglyceride levels is essential. By increasing your intake of fiber-rich foods, you can support better triglyceride management and overall heart health.

As we continue our journey toward a triglyceride-friendly diet, remember that small changes can have a significant impact. Incorporating fiber into your meals doesn't have to be complicated; it's about making informed choices and gradually building habits that support your health and well-being. In the chapters that follow, we'll explore more dietary strategies and practical tips to help you on your path to taming triglycerides.

CHAPTER 7

The Role of Exercise

In our ongoing exploration of taming high triglycerides through a holistic approach to health, we've covered various aspects of diet and nutrition. Now, in Chapter 7, we shift our focus to another critical component of a heart-healthy lifestyle – exercise. Physical activity is a powerful tool for managing triglycerides and promoting overall cardiovascular well-being. This chapter explores the role of exercise in triglyceride management, the types of exercise that are most effective, and practical tips for incorporating physical activity into your daily routine.

The Benefits of Exercise

Exercise is not just about burning calories and losing weight; it offers a multitude of benefits for heart health and triglyceride management:

1. **Lowering Triglycerides:** Regular physical activity can lower triglyceride levels, especially when combined with dietary changes.

Exercise helps your body use triglycerides for energy, reducing their presence in the bloodstream.

2. **Boosting "Good" Cholesterol:** Exercise can raise high-density lipoprotein (HDL) cholesterol, often referred to as "good" cholesterol. Higher levels of HDL can help remove excess triglycerides from the blood.

3. **Blood Sugar Control:** Physical activity enhances insulin sensitivity, helping your body regulate blood sugar levels. Stable blood

sugar levels are associated with lower triglyceride levels.

4. **Weight Management:** Exercise plays a crucial role in maintaining a healthy weight. Excess body weight is a significant contributor to elevated triglycerides.

5. **Reducing Inflammation:** Chronic inflammation is linked to heart disease and high triglycerides. Exercise can help reduce inflammation in the body.

6. **Strengthening the Heart:** Regular exercise strengthens the heart

muscle, improving its ability to pump blood efficiently.

Types of Exercise

The most effective exercise routines for managing triglycerides usually include a combination of cardiovascular (aerobic) and strength-training (anaerobic) exercises. Here's a closer look at each type:

1. **Cardiovascular (Aerobic) Exercise:** Cardio workouts get your heart rate up and improve the efficiency of your cardiovascular system.

They're excellent for lowering triglycerides and improving overall heart health. Some examples of aerobic exercises include:

- **Brisk Walking:** Walking at a pace that raises your heart rate.

- **Running:** A more intense form of aerobic exercise.

- **Cycling:** Riding a bicycle, either outdoors or on a stationary bike.

- **Swimming:** A full-body workout that's easy on the joints.

- **Dancing:** An enjoyable way to get your heart pumping.
- **Aerobics Classes:** Group classes that typically involve high-energy movements.

2. **Strength-Training (Anaerobic) Exercise:** Strength training builds muscle mass and boosts your metabolism, helping you burn more calories, even at rest. While it doesn't directly lower triglycerides, it supports overall weight management, which can impact triglyceride levels.

Examples of strength-training exercises include:

- **Weightlifting:** Using free weights or weight machines to target specific muscle groups.
- **Bodyweight Exercises:** Using your own body weight for resistance, such as push-ups, squats, and lunges.
- **Resistance Bands:** Stretchy bands that provide resistance for strength exercises.
- **Yoga and Pilates:** These practices

combine strength, flexibility, and balance.

Creating a Balanced Exercise Routine

A well-rounded exercise routine often combines both aerobic and anaerobic exercises for the best results. Here's how to create a balanced routine:

- **Cardiovascular Exercise:** Aim for at least 150 minutes of moderate-intensity aerobic activity or 75 minutes of vigorous-intensity aerobic activity per week, spread out over at least three days. This could be as simple as a 30-minute brisk walk most days of the week.

- **Strength Training:** Include strength-training exercises for all major muscle groups at least two days per week. You can work with free weights, resistance bands, or your body weight.
- **Flexibility and Balance:** Don't forget to incorporate flexibility and balance exercises, like yoga or stretching, to maintain joint health and prevent injuries.

- **Rest and Recovery:** Allow your body time to rest and recover between intense workouts to prevent overtraining and injury.

Practical Tips for Getting Started

Starting or restarting an exercise routine can be challenging, but the benefits for your triglycerides and overall health are well worth the effort. Here are some practical tips for getting started and staying motivated:

1. **Set Realistic Goals:** Start with achievable goals that

match your current fitness level. Gradually increase the intensity and duration of your workouts.

2. **Find Activities You Enjoy:** Choose activities you genuinely like, whether it's dancing, swimming, hiking, or gardening. If you enjoy the exercise, you're more likely to stick with it.

3. **Create a Schedule:** Plan your workouts and add them to your calendar as you would with other appointments. Consistency is key.

4. **Work with a Professional:** Consider working with a fitness trainer or physical therapist, especially if you're new to exercise or have specific health concerns.

5. **Stay Accountable:** Find an exercise buddy or join a fitness class or group to stay motivated and accountable.

6. **Listen to Your Body:** Pay attention to how your body feels during and after exercise. If you experience pain or discomfort, consult a healthcare professional.

7. **Track Your Progress:** Keep a workout journal or use a fitness app to track your progress and celebrate your achievements.

The Big Picture

Chapter 7 underscores the significant role that exercise plays in managing triglycerides and promoting heart health. Regular physical activity offers a multitude of benefits, including lower triglycerides, improved cholesterol profiles, blood sugar control, and weight management. By incorporating both aerobic and anaerobic exercises into your routine and staying committed to a balanced, heart-healthy lifestyle, you can make significant strides in taming high triglycerides.

Remember that every step you take towards a more active lifestyle contributes to better heart health. As we continue our journey to taming triglycerides in the chapters ahead, stay motivated, and keep moving towards your health and wellness goals.

CHAPTER 8

Lifestyle and Long-Term Triglyceride Management

As we approach the final chapter of our journey to tame high triglycerides through a holistic approach to health, we delve into the pivotal topic of lifestyle choices and their long-term impact on triglyceride management. While diet and exercise are crucial components, this chapter focuses on additional lifestyle factors that can significantly influence your triglyceride levels, including stress management, sleep, and avoiding harmful habits.

Stress Management

Stress has a profound impact on our physical and emotional well-being, and it can affect triglyceride levels as well. When we experience stress, our bodies release hormones like cortisol, which can lead to elevated triglycerides. Chronic stress can also trigger unhealthy coping mechanisms, such as overeating or making poor dietary choices. Here's how you can manage stress for better triglyceride control:

1. **Mindfulness and Relaxation Techniques:** Incorporate mindfulness practices like meditation, deep breathing exercises, or yoga into your daily routine. These practices can help reduce stress and promote emotional well-being.

2. **Physical Activity:** Regular exercise is not only beneficial for triglyceride management but also for stress reduction. Engaging in physical activity releases endorphins, which are natural mood lifters.

3. **Time Management:** Organize your daily tasks and prioritize what's most important. Managing your time efficiently can help reduce stress.

4. **Social Connections:** Maintain healthy relationships and a strong social support network. Talking to friends and loved ones can provide emotional relief during stressful times.

5. **Seek Professional Help:** If stress becomes overwhelming or chronic, consider consulting a mental

health professional for guidance and support.

Quality Sleep

Sleep is often undervalued but plays a crucial role in overall health, including triglyceride management. Poor sleep quality or insufficient sleep can disrupt hormonal balance and lead to higher triglyceride levels. To promote better sleep:

1. **Establish a Sleep Routine:** Go to bed and wake up at the same time every day, even on weekends.

2. **Create a Relaxing Bedtime Ritual:** Engage in calming activities before bed, such as reading, taking a warm bath, or practicing relaxation techniques.

3. **Limit Screen Time:** Avoid screens (phones, computers, TVs) at least an hour before bedtime, as the blue light emitted can interfere with your sleep-wake cycle.

4. **Create a Comfortable Sleep Environment:** Ensure your bedroom is cool, dark, and quiet. Invest in a comfortable mattress and pillows.

5. **Limit Caffeine and Alcohol:** Avoid caffeine and alcohol close to bedtime, as they can disrupt sleep patterns.

6. **Regular Exercise:** Engaging in regular physical activity can improve sleep quality. However, avoid intense exercise close to bedtime.

7. **Manage Stress:** Stress and anxiety can interfere with sleep. Incorporate stress management techniques into your daily routine to promote better sleep.

Avoiding Harmful Habits

Certain lifestyle habits can significantly impact triglycerides and overall heart health. Avoiding these harmful habits is essential for long-term triglyceride management:

1. **Smoking:** Smoking is a major risk factor for heart disease and can lead to elevated triglyceride levels. Quitting smoking is one of the best things you can do for your heart.
2. **Excessive Alcohol Consumption:** Drinking alcohol in excess can raise

triglyceride levels. If you choose to consume alcohol, do so in moderation, following recommended guidelines.

3. **Sugary and Processed Foods:** Highly processed foods and sugary beverages can contribute to elevated triglycerides. Minimize your intake of these items and opt for whole, unprocessed foods.

4. **Sedentary Lifestyle:** Physical inactivity is a risk factor for high triglycerides and heart disease. Aim for regular physical activity to

support triglyceride management.

Long-Term Triglyceride Management

Managing high triglycerides is not a short-term endeavor; it's about making sustainable lifestyle changes for the long haul. Here are some strategies for maintaining healthy triglyceride levels over time:

1. **Regular Monitoring:** Keep track of your triglyceride levels through regular check-ups with your healthcare provider. This

can help you stay on top of your progress and make necessary adjustments.

2. **Lifelong Nutrition:** Continue to prioritize a heart-healthy diet rich in fruits, vegetables, lean proteins, and whole grains. Be mindful of portion sizes and limit saturated and trans fats.

3. **Consistent Exercise:** Make physical activity a regular part of your life. Aim for a balanced combination of aerobic and strength-training exercises.

4. **Stress Resilience:** Practice stress management techniques consistently, even when you're not feeling particularly stressed. This proactive approach can help prevent stress-related triglyceride spikes.

5. **Quality Sleep:** Prioritize sleep hygiene and ensure you consistently get the recommended amount of sleep for your age.

6. **Habitual Health:** Avoid harmful habits like smoking and excessive alcohol consumption. Substitute

these behaviors with healthier alternatives.

7. **Regular Healthcare Visits:** Continue to see your healthcare provider for routine check-ups and screenings. These visits are essential for early detection and intervention if necessary.

The Big Picture

Chapter 8 underscores the importance of long-term lifestyle choices in maintaining healthy triglyceride levels. While dietary changes and exercise are vital components, factors like stress management, sleep quality, and avoiding harmful habits contribute significantly to your overall heart health.

Remember that managing triglycerides is a continuous journey that requires commitment and consistency. By adopting a holistic approach to health and making informed choices, you can take control of your triglyceride levels and enjoy better heart health for years to come.

CHAPTER 9

Monitoring and Maintaining Your Triglycerides

As we approach the final chapter of our journey to manage high triglycerides through a holistic approach to health, we come to a pivotal phase - ongoing monitoring and maintenance. This chapter focuses on how to keep track of your triglyceride levels and maintain the progress you've made through diet, exercise, lifestyle changes, and medications, if necessary. It's about ensuring that your efforts lead to long-term health and well-being.

The Importance of Monitoring

Regular monitoring of your triglyceride levels is crucial for several reasons:

1. **Assessing Progress:** Monitoring allows you to track how your efforts to lower triglycerides are working. You can see if your dietary changes, exercise routine, and lifestyle

adjustments are making a positive impact.

2. **Early Detection:** It helps detect any fluctuations or increases in triglyceride levels early on, which can be addressed promptly to prevent further complications.

3. **Medication Management:** If you're on medication to control triglycerides, monitoring helps ensure that your treatment plan is effective. Your healthcare provider can adjust your medications if needed.

4. **Motivation:** Seeing improvements in your triglyceride levels can motivate you to stay on track with your healthy lifestyle choices.

Frequency of Monitoring

The frequency of triglyceride monitoring varies from person to person and depends on your initial levels, overall health, and the effectiveness of your triglyceride-lowering strategies. Generally, you can expect:

1. **Regular Check-Ups:** Your healthcare provider may

recommend monitoring your triglycerides as part of your routine check-ups. This could be annually or more frequently if you have higher risk factors.

2. **After Medication Changes:** If you're prescribed medication, your healthcare provider may request more frequent testing initially to evaluate the medication's effectiveness.

3. **During Significant Lifestyle Changes:** If you make significant changes to your diet, exercise, or other

lifestyle factors, monitoring your triglycerides can help assess the impact of these changes.

Maintaining Your Progress

Maintaining healthy triglyceride levels is about more than just lowering them initially; it's about sustaining your progress over the long term. Here's how to ensure your efforts lead to lasting benefits:

1. **Consistency:** Keep up with the dietary changes, exercise routine, and lifestyle adjustments that have

proven effective in lowering your triglycerides.

2. **Regular Follow-Ups:** Continue to see your healthcare provider for regular check-ups and follow their recommendations for monitoring.

3. **Stay Informed:** Stay informed about the latest research and guidelines regarding triglycerides and heart health. This knowledge can help you make informed decisions about your lifestyle.

4. **Adaptability:** Be prepared to adapt your approach if

necessary. Lifestyle factors, health conditions, and medications may change over time, and your triglyceride management plan may need to evolve accordingly.

Medications and Triglyceride Management

In some cases, lifestyle changes alone may not be sufficient to manage high triglycerides, and medication may be necessary. Medications can be a crucial part of your triglyceride-lowering strategy, especially if you have very high levels or other risk factors for heart disease.

Common medications used to lower triglycerides include:

1. **Statins:** These drugs are primarily used to lower LDL cholesterol but can also have a modest effect on triglycerides.

2. **Fibrates:** Fibrates are specifically designed to lower triglycerides and raise HDL cholesterol. They can be used alone or in combination with other medications.

3. **Omega-3 Fatty Acids:** Prescription omega-3 fatty acid medications, such as Lovaza, can help lower triglycerides, particularly in people with very high levels.

4. **Niacin (Vitamin B3):** Niacin can lower triglycerides and raise HDL cholesterol but may have side effects and is typically used when other medications are not effective.

5. **Bile Acid Sequestrants:** These drugs can lower LDL cholesterol and may have a

modest effect on triglycerides.

6. **Newer Medications:** Some newer medications, such as PCSK9 inhibitors, are used primarily for lowering LDL cholesterol but may also have some impact on triglycerides.

Working with Your Healthcare Provider

Your healthcare provider is a crucial partner in your journey to manage triglycerides effectively. Here are some tips for collaborating effectively:

1. **Open Communication:** Be open and honest about your lifestyle, dietary habits, exercise routine, and any medications or supplements you're taking.

2. **Ask Questions:** Don't hesitate to ask questions about your triglyceride levels, treatment options, and any concerns you may have.

3. **Follow Recommendations:** Follow your healthcare provider's recommendations regarding diet, exercise,

medications, and monitoring.

4. **Keep Records:** Keep a record of your triglyceride levels, medications, and any changes to your lifestyle. This can help both you and your provider track your progress.

5. **Discuss Side Effects:** If you experience any side effects from medications, inform your healthcare provider promptly. They can adjust your treatment plan if necessary.

The Big Picture

Chapter 9 underscores the importance of ongoing monitoring and maintenance in managing high triglycerides. Your journey doesn't end when you achieve healthy triglyceride levels; it continues with consistent efforts to sustain those levels for the long term. Regular monitoring, lifestyle consistency, and effective collaboration with your healthcare provider are keys to maintaining your progress and enjoying lasting heart health benefits.

Remember that managing triglycerides is a holistic endeavor, encompassing diet, exercise, stress management, and other lifestyle choices. By staying proactive, informed, and committed, you can successfully navigate this journey towards better heart health and overall well-being.

CHAPTER 10

Celebrating Success and Looking Forward

Congratulations! You've completed the journey to manage high triglycerides through a comprehensive approach to health. As we wrap up our exploration, Chapter 10 is a celebration of your achievements and a reflection on the road ahead. It's a time to appreciate your progress, acknowledge the positive changes you've made, and set the stage for a healthy, fulfilling future.

Celebrating Your Success

Taking control of your triglycerides and improving your heart health is a significant accomplishment. It's important to celebrate your success, no matter how big or small. Here are some ways to acknowledge your achievements:

1. **Reflect on Your Journey:** Take a moment to reflect on the changes you've made in your life, from dietary improvements to

embracing regular exercise. Recognize the determination and effort you've invested in your health.

2. **Celebrate Milestones:** Consider marking important milestones along the way. Whether it's a specific weight loss goal, reaching your exercise targets, or consistently maintaining healthy triglyceride levels, celebrate these accomplishments.

3. **Share Your Success:** Share your journey and success with friends and loved ones. Your story may

inspire others to take control of their health as well.

4. **Treat Yourself:** It's okay to reward yourself for your hard work. Treat yourself to something special, like a day at the spa, a favorite meal, or a new book.

5. **Positive Self-Talk:** Practice positive self-talk and acknowledge your efforts regularly. Encouraging words and self-compassion can boost your motivation.

Maintaining Your Progress

While it's essential to celebrate your achievements, it's equally crucial to maintain the progress you've made. Here's how to continue on your path to better heart health:

1. **Consistency:** Keep up with the healthy habits you've developed, whether it's your improved diet, regular exercise routine, stress management techniques, or medication regimen.

2. **Regular Monitoring:** Stay engaged with your healthcare provider and continue to monitor your

triglyceride levels. Regular check-ups help detect any changes early and allow for timely adjustments.

3. **Stay Informed:** Keep yourself informed about the latest research and recommendations in cardiovascular health. Being knowledgeable empowers you to make informed decisions about your lifestyle and treatment options.

4. **Adaptability:** Be open to adapting your approach as needed. Life is full of changes, and your health needs may evolve over time.

Flexibility is key to long-term success.

5. **Community Support:** Stay connected with your support network. Engage in discussions, share your experiences, and seek advice from others who are on similar health journeys.

Setting New Goals

With your achievements as a foundation, it's time to set new goals for your health and well-being. Goal-setting keeps you motivated and provides direction for your continued growth. Here's how to establish new objectives:

1. **Assess Your Priorities:**
Consider what aspects of
your health and life are most
important to you. These
might include maintaining
healthy triglyceride levels,
achieving a specific fitness
goal, or enhancing your
overall well-being.

2. **SMART Goals:** Create
SMART (Specific,
Measurable, Achievable,
Relevant, Time-Bound)
goals that are clear and
realistic. For example,
instead of setting a vague
goal like "exercise more,"
specify a goal like "walk for

30 minutes five days a week."

3. **Break It Down:** Divide larger goals into smaller, manageable steps. This makes them less daunting and easier to track.

4. **Track Your Progress:** Keep a journal or use an app to track your progress toward your goals. Celebrate each step you achieve along the way.

5. **Stay Accountable:** Share your goals with someone who can help hold you accountable, whether it's a

friend, family member, or healthcare provider.

The Future of Heart Health

As you look forward to the future, it's essential to recognize that managing high triglycerides is a lifelong commitment to heart health. Here are some key considerations for your ongoing journey:

1. **A Lifetime of Health:** Embrace the idea that the habits you've cultivated are not temporary measures but lifelong choices. Sustainable

changes are more likely to yield lasting benefits.

2. **Age-Related Considerations:** As you age, your health needs may change. Regular check-ups and discussions with your healthcare provider will help you adapt your approach to meet these evolving needs.

3. **Support Systems:** Continue to lean on your support network. Friends, family, healthcare providers, and support groups can provide encouragement and guidance.

4. **Explore New Horizons:** Be open to exploring new aspects of health and wellness. This might include trying different forms of exercise, exploring new dietary options, or delving into stress-reduction techniques.

5. **Advocacy for Heart Health:** Consider becoming an advocate for heart health in your community. Sharing your story and knowledge can inspire and educate others.

The Big Picture

Chapter 10 is a time of celebration, reflection, and anticipation. Your journey to manage high triglycerides has been a transformative experience that has brought positive changes to your life. As you celebrate your success, remember that your health journey is ongoing, and the choices you make today will impact your future well-being.

By staying committed to your health, setting new goals, and embracing the principles of a heart-healthy lifestyle, you can look forward to a future filled with vitality, well-being, and the satisfaction of knowing that you've taken charge of your heart health.

CONCLUSION

A Heart-Healthy Journey to Tame High Triglycerides

In the pages of this book, we've embarked on a transformative journey—a journey to understand, manage, and conquer high triglycerides through a holistic approach to health. We've explored the intricate web of factors that contribute to elevated triglyceride levels and, more importantly, the powerful tools and strategies available to bring them under control.

Our journey began with a deep dive into the world of triglycerides, unraveling the science behind these fatty molecules that play a crucial role in our cardiovascular health. We uncovered their connection to heart disease, diabetes, and other health conditions, highlighting why it's so essential to manage them effectively.

From there, we ventured into the heart of our dietary choices, discovering how what we eat can significantly impact triglyceride levels. We explored the Mediterranean diet, the DASH diet, and other heart-healthy eating plans that have the potential to transform our health from the inside out. We learned how to decipher nutrition labels, make wise choices in the grocery store, and cook up delicious, triglyceride-friendly meals in our own kitchens.

Exercise took center stage in Chapter 7, where we delved into the profound influence of physical activity on our cardiovascular well-being. We recognized that regular exercise is not just about shedding pounds; it's about strengthening our hearts, lowering triglycerides, and enhancing our overall quality of life.

Chapter 8 underscored the importance of managing stress, getting quality sleep, and steering clear of harmful habits. We discovered that nurturing our mental and emotional well-being is as critical as nourishing our bodies with the right foods and activities.

In Chapter 9, we learned the value of consistent monitoring and maintenance, recognizing that our journey doesn't end when we achieve our health goals. Regular check-ups with healthcare providers, ongoing self-assessment, and adaptability are the cornerstones of sustainable triglyceride management.

And finally, in Chapter 10, we celebrated our achievements, recognized the importance of maintaining our progress, and set new, inspiring goals for our health and well-being. We looked ahead to a future filled with vitality and the satisfaction of knowing that we've taken charge of our heart health.

As we conclude this book, remember that managing high triglycerides is not just a duty; it's an act of self-love and self-preservation. Your health is a precious gift, and by taking the knowledge you've gained here and translating it into action, you're investing in a future of well-being and vitality.

Your journey doesn't end with these pages; it's a lifelong expedition filled with opportunities for growth, discovery, and empowerment. Your heart is in your hands, and you have the tools, knowledge, and determination to keep it healthy for years to come.

So, go forth with confidence and courage. Embrace the principles of a heart-healthy lifestyle, seek support and guidance when needed, and never forget that you have the power to shape your health destiny. This is not just the end of a book; it's the beginning of a healthier, happier you.